THE DANGERS OF
MARIJUANA

JODYANNE BENSON

PowerKiDS
press
New York

Published in 2020 by The Rosen Publishing Group, Inc.
29 East 21st Street, New York, NY 10010

First Edition

Editor: Jenna Tolli
Book Design: Reann Nye

Photo Credits: Cover gradyreese/E+/Getty Images; series art patpitchaya/Shutterstock.com; p. 4 Joshua Rainey Photography/Shutterstock.com; p. 5 Canna Obscura/Shutterstock.com; p. 7 OpenRangeStock/Shutterstock.com; p. 9 Africa Studio/Shutterstock.com; p. 11 uzhursky/Shutterstock.com; p. 13 SeventyFour/Shutterstock.com; p. 15 Sherry Yates Young/Shutterstock.com; p. 16 designer491/Shutterstock.com; p. 17 pixelheadphoto digitalskillet/Shutterstock.com; p. 19 Jasmin Merdan/ Moment/ Getty Images; p. 21 Photographee.eu/Shutterstock.com; p. 22 Brocreative/Shutterstock.com.

Cataloging-in-Publication Data

Names: Benson, Jodyanne.
Title: The dangers of marijuana / Jodyanne Benson.
Description: New York : PowerKids Press, 2020. | Series: The dangers of drugs, alcohol, and smoking | Includes glossary and index.
Identifiers: ISBN 9781725309784 (pbk.) | ISBN 9781725309807 (library bound) | ISBN 9781725309791 (6 pack)
Subjects: LCSH: Marijuana–Juvenile literature. | Marijuana abuse–Juvenile literature.
Classification: LCC HV5822.M3 B46 2020 | DDC 362.29'5–dc23

Manufactured in the United States of America

Some of the images in this book illustrate individuals who are models. The depictions do not imply actual situations or events.

CPSIA Compliance Information: Batch #CWPK20. For Further Information contact Rosen Publishing, New York, New York at 1-800-237-9932.

CONTENTS

MARIJUANA EVERYWHERE

What is marijuana? Why do people smoke marijuana? Is marijuana safe? You may have wondered about these questions. You may have even seen advertisements for marijuana. That's because this drug or types of it are **legal** in parts of the United States.

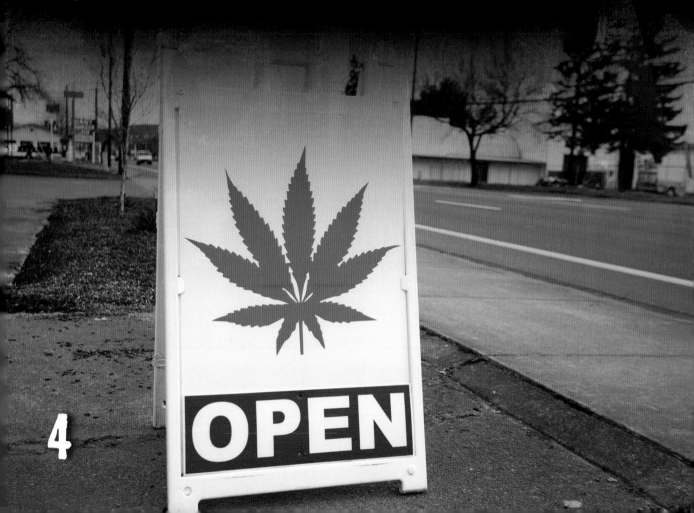

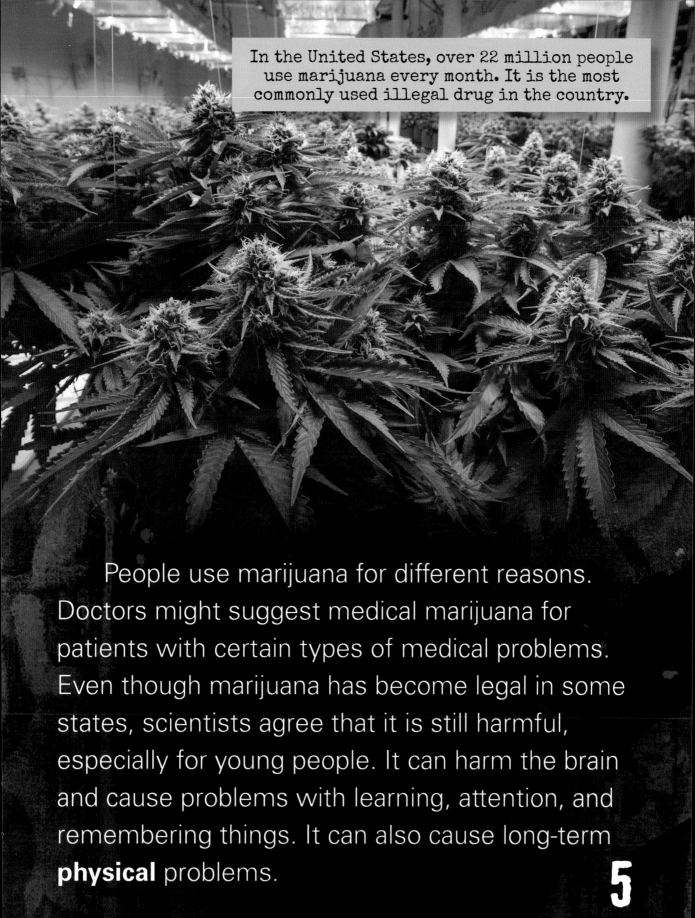

In the United States, over 22 million people use marijuana every month. It is the most commonly used illegal drug in the country.

People use marijuana for different reasons. Doctors might suggest medical marijuana for patients with certain types of medical problems. Even though marijuana has become legal in some states, scientists agree that it is still harmful, especially for young people. It can harm the brain and cause problems with learning, attention, and remembering things. It can also cause long-term **physical** problems.

WHAT IS MARIJUANA?

Marijuana is a mixture of the dried flowers and leaves from the cannabis plant. You may have heard it called weed, pot, grass, Mary Jane, or dope. Marijuana is rolled and smoked like a cigarette, put in cigars or pipes, mixed with food, or made into tea.

There is a chemical in marijuana called THC, which is produced by the plant's leaves and buds. It's a mind-altering chemical, which means that it changes the way you think and act. There are also **synthetic** cannabinoids, which are made by people. Sometimes these are called synthetic marijuana. They are very strong and unsafe.

DANGER ZONE

Recently, people have also started to inhale, or breathe in, marijuana using vaporizers. These are small, electronic devices that are filled with oil from marijuana plants. This is called vaping.

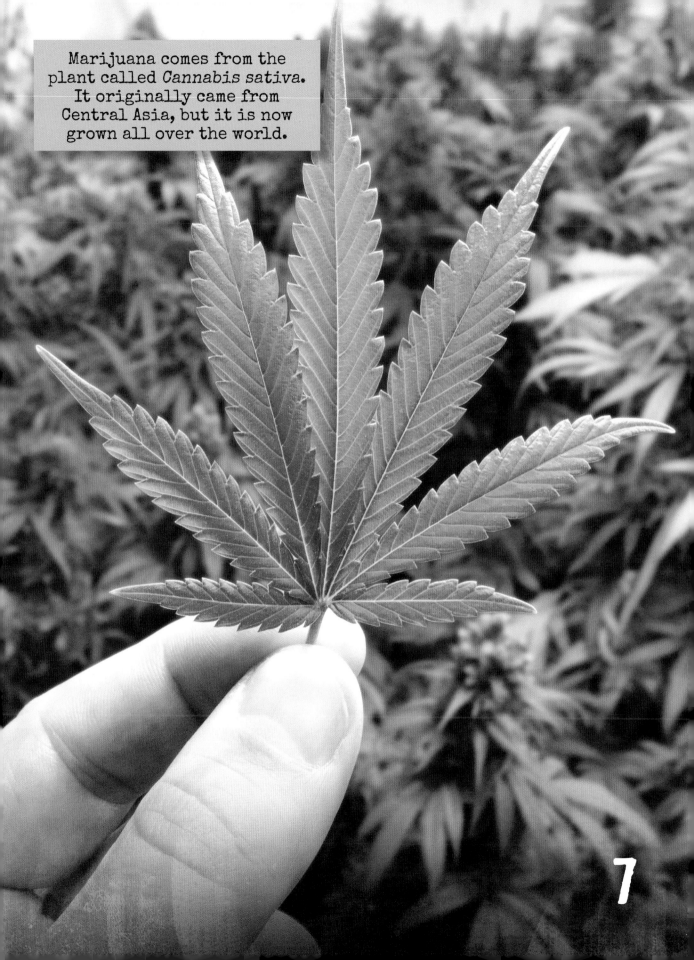

Marijuana comes from the plant called *Cannabis sativa*. It originally came from Central Asia, but it is now grown all over the world.

7

THE HISTORY OF MARIJUANA

Marijuana has been used by people around the world for a long time. **Evidence** has been found that ancient societies used the drug for medicine. These early plants had very low amounts of THC. This means they would not have had the mind-altering effects we see today.

However, these ancient societies may have known that the cannabis plant could change how the mind works. They may have also grown plants with higher THC levels to use in religious **ceremonies**. Burned cannabis seeds have been found in graves in China and Siberia that date all the way back to 500 BC.

DANGER ZONE

Foods and drinks with marijuana in them have some different risks than smoking marijuana. There is an even higher risk of poisoning.

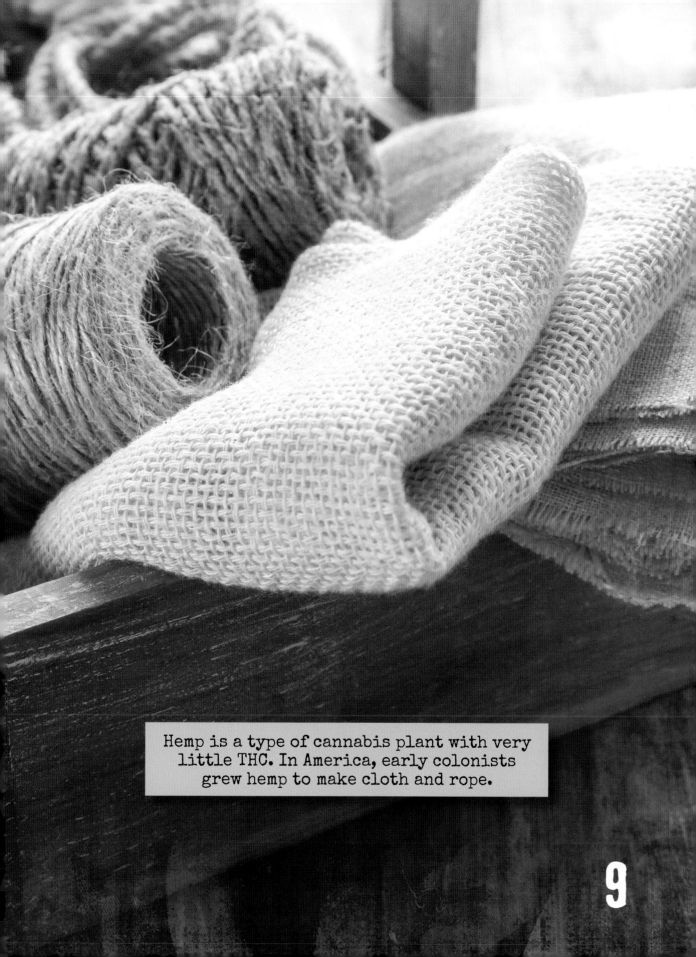

Hemp is a type of cannabis plant with very little THC. In America, early colonists grew hemp to make cloth and rope.

EFFECTS OF MARIJUANA

When people smoke marijuana, THC and other chemicals go into their lungs and blood. Then the blood moves those chemicals through the body and to the brain, which makes people feel happy and relaxed. Sometimes people see things differently after smoking marijuana, like brighter colors. It can also make them feel hungry and cause them to laugh more.

Marijuana also has many harmful effects. It can cause someone to become nervous and scared. People who have taken a lot of marijuana may **hallucinate** or forget who they are. Using a lot of marijuana has been linked to serious mental health problems, which are related to how we think, feel, and act.

DANGER ZONE

The amount of THC in marijuana has gone up in recent years. Higher THC levels make it more likely that those using it will have a bad response to the drug.

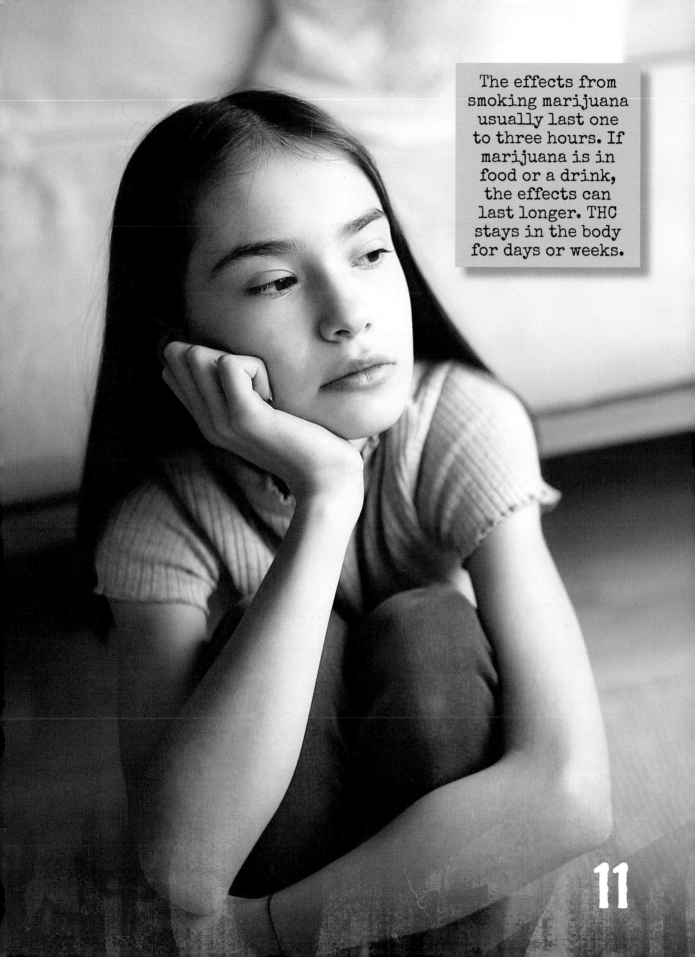

The effects from smoking marijuana usually last one to three hours. If marijuana is in food or a drink, the effects can last longer. THC stays in the body for days or weeks.

11

DANGERS FOR YOUNG PEOPLE

Marijuana is a harmful drug. It immediately affects the brain and body. THC in marijuana causes problems with thinking, problem-solving, learning, and memory. It can also make people feel light-headed or tired. This makes it very dangerous, or unsafe, to drive or do other activities after using marijuana.

There are also more long-lasting side effects. Marijuana hurts certain parts of the brain. It can harm the lungs and make it harder to breathe. This drug also makes it harder for the body to fight infections, which are sicknesses caused by germs. People who use marijuana a lot can become more nervous, sad, and afraid.

DANGER ZONE

Marijuana is especially dangerous for children and teenagers. Marijuana use can lead to changes in their brains, which are still growing.

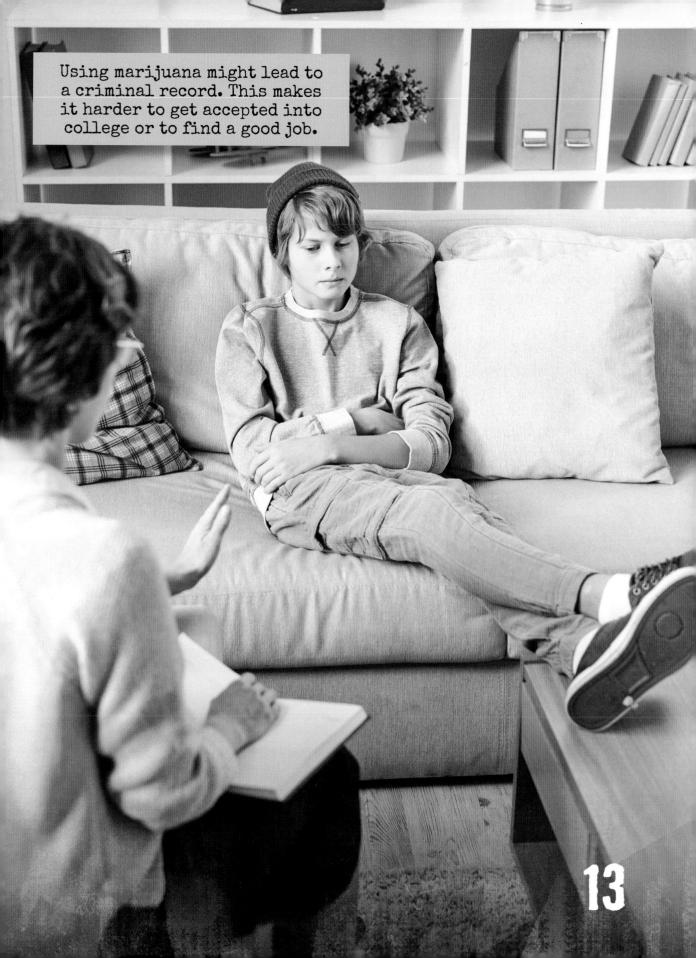

Using marijuana might lead to a criminal record. This makes it harder to get accepted into college or to find a good job.

13

MEDICAL MARIJUANA

The marijuana plant is sometimes used to help sick people feel better. This is called medical marijuana. The United States government has not approved the plant itself as medicine. The government tries to make sure that medicine is safe before people use it. Still, scientists have found that certain chemicals in marijuana called cannabinoids can benefit some people. So far, the government has approved two medications with cannabinoids.

Scientists continue to study how chemicals in marijuana can help to treat different **symptoms**. For example, cannabinoids can help people eat again after being sick. They can also help with pain, swelling, and muscle control problems.

DANGER ZONE

There are still risks and side effects for using medical marijuana. Doctors work with patients to decide if using this drug is right for them.

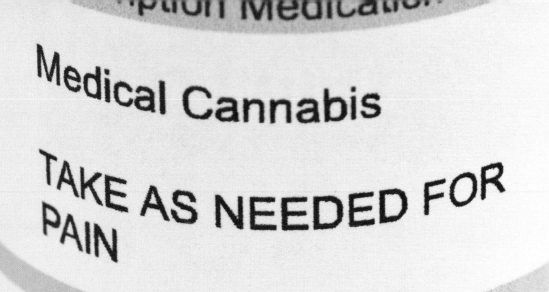

ption Medication

Medical Cannabis

TAKE AS NEEDED FOR PAIN

30 CT

No Refill

More studies are needed to understand the long-term side effects for patients that use medical marijuana, especially for older adults and people with serious illnesses.

LEGAL OR NOT?

Marijuana has been a big topic in the news. Some states have made marijuana legal to use, but this doesn't mean that it's always safe.

Marijuana is legal in some states, but it is illegal under **federal** law. More studies are needed for the federal government to decide if the benefits are higher than the risks.

FEDERAL AND STATE MARIJUANA LAWS

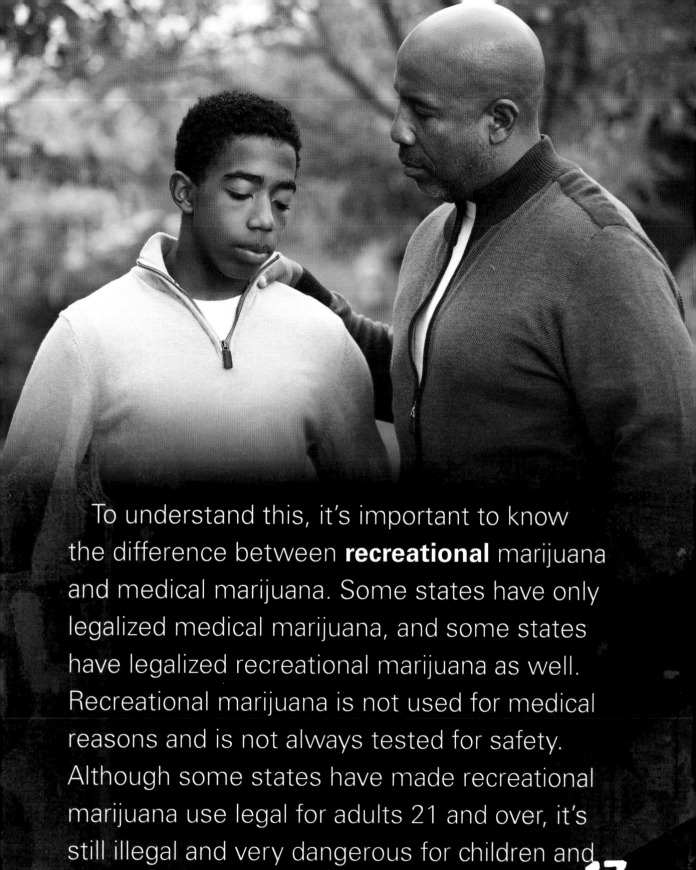

To understand this, it's important to know the difference between **recreational** marijuana and medical marijuana. Some states have only legalized medical marijuana, and some states have legalized recreational marijuana as well. Recreational marijuana is not used for medical reasons and is not always tested for safety. Although some states have made recreational marijuana use legal for adults 21 and over, it's still illegal and very dangerous for children and teenagers to use.

17

ADDICTION

Marijuana use can lead to a marijuana abuse disorder, which is a medical illness. When someone has this disorder, they can't stop using the drug even though it is causing serious problems. Between 9 to 30 percent of people who use the drug often can develop a marijuana abuse disorder. People with very serious abuse disorders could become addicted.

People who use marijuana and want to give it up often become very sick. This is called withdrawal. They can become angry, sad, worried, and scared. They also have trouble sleeping and cannot eat very well. There are no medications to treat this disorder, but other kinds of support can help.

DANGER ZONE

People who start using marijuana before they are 18 are four to seven times more likely than adults to develop a marijuana abuse disorder.

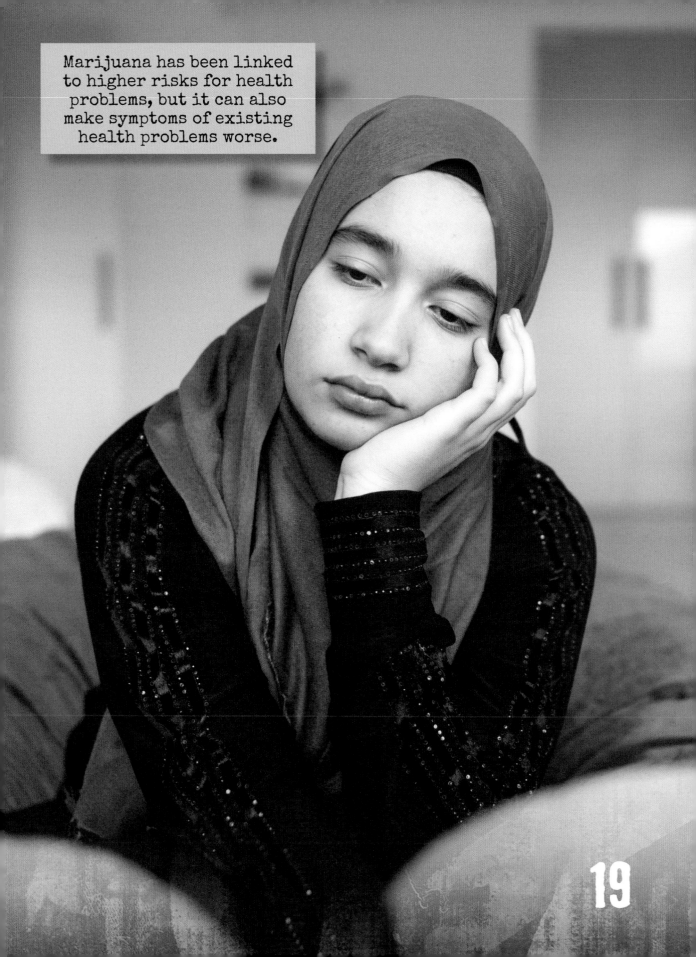

Marijuana has been linked to higher risks for health problems, but it can also make symptoms of existing health problems worse.

FINDING HELP

Do you know someone who is using marijuana? There are different types of **treatment** and ways to help. First, it's important to talk to someone you trust, like a parent or teacher.

Counseling can help people with a marijuana abuse disorder or an addiction to marijuana. During counseling, people talk openly about how they feel. There are also support groups where people who are addicted to marijuana meet and help each other quit. Finally, it's very helpful for family and friends to learn about the dangers of marijuana and teach others how it can be harmful.

Getting help for a disorder or addiction is the best way to get on the right path. There are many ways to get help, like talking to a counselor.

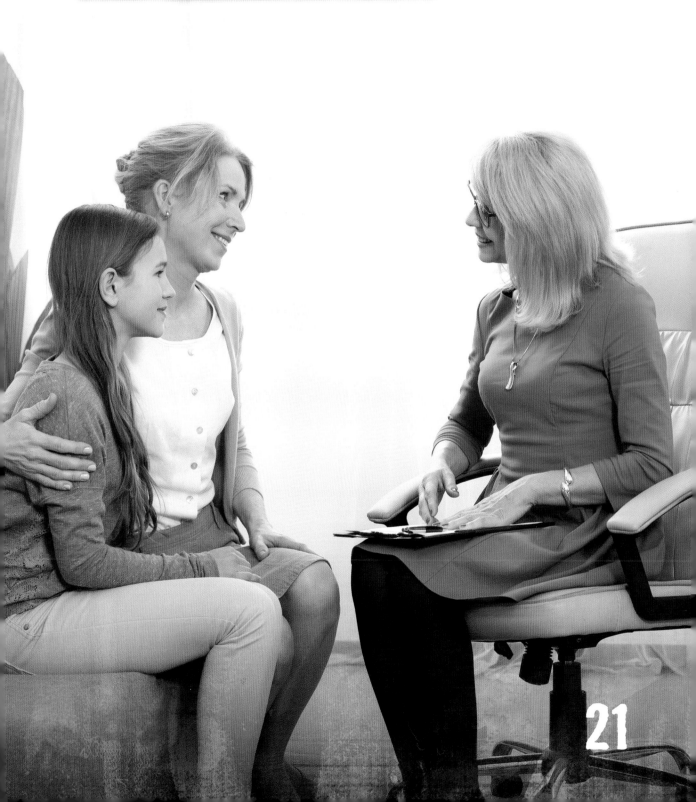

MAKING GOOD CHOICES

There are many dangerous effects from using marijuana. It can hurt your body and brain. Students who use marijuana are more likely to get lower grades and drop out of school. It can also lead to serious mental and emotional problems. In states where marijuana is not legal, it can even lead to a criminal record.

You can decide what your **future** will look like by making good choices today. By understanding the dangers of marijuana and other drugs, you can choose to make smart decisions—including staying away from trying them.

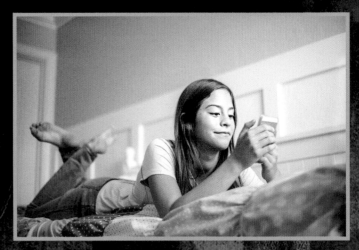

GLOSSARY

ceremonies: Formal acts or events that are part of a social or religious occasion.

counseling: Advice and support given to someone to help them with a problem.

evidence: Something that shows that something else is true.

federal: Relating to the central government of the United States.

future: The period of time after the present time.

hallucinate: To see or feel something that is not really there.

legal: Allowed by the law.

physical: Relating to the body.

recreational: Done for pleasure instead of medical reasons.

symptom: A change in the body or mind that shows something bad.

synthetic: Made by combining different substances that are not natural.

treatment: Medical care given to a patient for an illness or injury.

INDEX

WEBSITES

Due to the changing nature of Internet links, PowerKids Press has developed an online list of websites related to the subject of this book. This site is updated regularly. Please use this link to access the list: www.powerkidslinks.com/das/marijuana